Ketogenic Diet

The Easiest Way to Lose Weight Fast for Beginners with Low-Carb, High-Fat Keto Clarity Diet.

I0422178

Introduction

Do you want to lose weight fast enough for a special event? Are you eager to jump-start weight loss so that you can get motivated? You might like to consider the ketogenic diet!

The keto diet is an extremely low carb and high fat diet that takes advantage of *ketosis,* which is a state that causes the body to burn stored fat. To trigger ketosis, one must eliminate carbohydrates and start consuming fat to train the body to burn fat instead of glucose for energy. This might seem like a dream come true, but it is quite a challenging diet to follow.

The good news is that this book will guide you through the keto diet. You will find a 7 day keto meal plan to make things easy for you, along with the recipes for each meal of the day. All the recipes call for cheap and healthy ingredients that are guaranteed to give you energy and designed to bring your body into a state of ketosis.

Enjoy the benefits of a strong and lean body. The keto diet can help you to lose weight, gain more energy, and improve your overall health.

Chapter 1 - What is the Keto Diet?

Okay, so everyone who has experienced dieting in the past knows all too well that eating carbs is bad for you, but did you know that eliminating carbs AND eating more fat will actually help you achieve weight loss? That is the premise of the keto diet.

Before you start stuffing yourself with butter and bacon, consider first the danger of high cholesterol levels and the chance of increasing your risk of developing heart disease. Try not to follow in the footsteps of Robert Atkins, the famous creator of the Atkins diet (a low carb, high fat and high protein diet), who, ironically, died of cardiac arrest. This is not what you want to achieve in the keto diet, certainly, which is why you should take precautionary measures before starting.

First of all, you need to know how the keto diet works. Basically, it triggers the liver to create ketosis. This is known as the state of ketosis, and it is the body's natural way to combat low glucose by enabling these ketones to break stored fat down for energy. Yes, that's right. Your own body will burn its stored fat.

The only way for ketosis to happen is to stop the body from producing glucose and insulin. To achieve this, you must starve your body of carbohydrates, which is the main source for glucose. This means, for the keto diet to work, you must restrain yourself from eating carbs, otherwise you will only be eating a lot of fat *and* carbs, which will then lead to even more weight gain. Sugar is included in this category, because it is also a source of glucose.

Getting rid of carbs from your diet is no easy feat, especially now when it seems to surround you everywhere you go. If you have been so used to eating carbs on a regular basis, the diet gets even more challenging because you will have carb and sugar cravings each time you refrain from eating them. It takes a certain amount of effort and determination on your part to make the decision to say no carbs. If you want results then you have to make certain sacrifices. Don't worry, for the results are certainly worth it all.

Those who have existing medical conditions such as diabetes and heart disease need to consult their doctor before they engage in this type of diet. In fact, anyone who wants to make changes to their regular diets should first talk to a medical professional to avoid problems. It is best that you take that approach as well.

So, how do you achieve a healthy balance of following the low carb and high fat keto diet without tragically falling ill? Plan your meals ahead and choose the right ingredients. While the recipes in this book do contain the typical keto diet meals, these should not be the bulk on your plate. What should make up at least half of your plate on every meal is steamed low carb vegetables.

Why vegetables, and why steamed?

Vegetables are actually a lot more delicious than most people think. On top of that, they are incredibly nutritious and high in fiber, both of which are necessary to help support a healthy and lean body. Locally produced, in season and organic vegetables are cheaper than most meals, in fact. You should visit your local farmers' market and grocery store and make inquiries.

The best way to ensure food safety is by submitting food to heat, and steaming is the best way to do that without causing the vegetables to lose most of their nutritional value.

Here are some suggested low carb vegetables that you should start consuming on a regular basis. Make sure to eat more than one type of vegetable if you want to get different kinds of vitamins and minerals each day:

- Spinach

- Green cabbage

- Cauliflower

- Romaine lettuce

- Bok choy

- Kale

- Collard Greens

- Green beans

In the keto diet, you should aim for approximately 5 percent of carbs, 25 percent of protein, and 70 percent of fats in all of your diet. Your fats should be poly-saturated, which you can get from olive and coconut oils, lean protein such as chicken and seafood, and nuts. If you want to hit two birds with one stone, then drizzle some extra virgin olive oil on your steamed low carb veggies and add your favorite natural seasonings.

Now that's easy keto!

On a similar note, you should beware of trans fats. You should avoid trans fats like the plague! These are the *fake* fats responsible for heart disease. Food fried in unnatural oils (those hydrogenated oils and other oils with multiple ingredients you cannot seem to pronounce correctly), margarine, and even butter contain a lot of fats. It is for this reason that the recipes in this book call only for grass fed butter. You should also minimize consumption of red meat. Even though this is originally part of the keto diet, large quantities of it will still increase your risk of heart disease and other illnesses. The best advice would be to always choose organic meat. Since these are expensive, you are likely to eat less and savor each bite more. Besides, they are guaranteed to be safer for your health.

Another highly crucial aspect when following the keto diet is to exercise every day. You read that right, every single day! You need to find a way to maximize the ketosis by letting those ketones burn up your fat as much as your body can take it. It does not even have to be high intensity exercise. A 30-minute power walk is enough to get you started. If your health allows it, engage in cardio and strength exercises at least 45 minutes every other day because these workouts will really enable your body to use up a lot of energy. Ideally, you should go to the gym and have a fitness instructor help you out, but if that is not possible for you then you should go online and search for as many workout videos as you can. It does not really matter where you exercise because the important thing is you are expending all of that energy!

Chapter 2 - The Keto Diet 7 Day Meal Plan

This 7-day keto diet plan will do all of the heavy lifting for you in the first week of the keto diet. All you need to do is to read the recipes that are called for each day in advance and prepare the ingredients based on the number of servings that you want.

You may cook in bulk and freeze the dishes, if it allows it, so you have enough food to last you for an entire week. Do not hesitate to put your own spin on each recipe by changing some of the ingredients (as long as they are still approved in the keto diet). Most importantly, do not forget to include a serving of low carb vegetables with every single dish!

Day 1:

Breakfast: Keto Popovers

Lunch: Tuna and Zucchini Roll-ups

Dinner: Sweet and Spicy Meatballs

Snack: Coconut and Cinnamon Balls

Day 2:

Breakfast: Pumpkin French Toast

Lunch: Bell Pepper and Chicken Kebabs

Dinner: Leftover Bell Pepper and Chicken Kebabs and Basic Bone Broth

Snack: Coconut and Cinnamon Balls

Day 3:

Breakfast: Cheesy Pancakes

Lunch: Pork and Mushroom Meatballs

Dinner: Simple Seafood Soup

Snack: Chocolate Mint Bars

Day 4:

Breakfast: Smoked Salmon Quiche

Lunch: Cheese Chicken Sticks

Dinner: Slow Cooked Kelp Noodle Pesto

Snack: Chocolate Mint Bars

Day 5:

Breakfast: Special Raspberry Waffles

Lunch: Basic Bone Broth and Cauliflower Bites

Dinner: Baked Scampi

Snack: Butter Pumpkin Balls

Day 6:

Breakfast: Baked Eggs on Avocado

Lunch: Tuna Salad

Dinner: Spaghetti Bolognese

Snack: Coconut and Blueberry Mini Cakes

Day 7:

Breakfast: Keto Popovers

Lunch: Leftover Spaghetti Bolognese

Dinner: Pork and Mushroom Meatballs with Kimchi

Snack: Mocha and Vanilla Butter Pops

Chapter 3 - Breakfast

Keto Popovers

Makes: 6 servings

Ingredients:

- ❖ 1/2 cup unflavored or vanilla whey protein powder
- ❖ 2 Tbsp melted coconut oil
- ❖ 2 eggs
- ❖ 1 cup unsweetened almond milk
- ❖ 1/4 tsp sea salt

Instructions:

1. Preheat the oven to 425 degrees F. Coat popover tins using nonstick cooking spray. Put the tins inside the oven and allow to heat up for about 5 minutes.

2. In the meantime, whisk together the eggs, protein powder, salt, and almond milk until well combined.

3. With mittens on, take the hot tins out of the oven and divide the coconut oil evenly among the tins. After that, fill each tin up to two-thirds full with the batter.

4. Bake for 15 minutes, then set the oven heat down to 235 degrees F. Bake for an extra 10 minutes or until puffed up.

5. Carefully remove from the oven and set on a wire rack to cool slightly before serving.

Pumpkin French Toast

Makes: 2 slices

Ingredients:

- ❖ 2 slices protein bread
- ❖ 1 Tbsp heavy cream
- ❖ 1 small egg
- ❖ 1 Tbsp grass fed butter
- ❖ 1/4 tsp vanilla extract
- ❖ Pumpkin pie spice

Instructions:

1. Place the protein bread on a plate and leave out overnight to dry.

2. In the morning, whisk the egg in a bowl and add a dash of pumpkin pie spice and the extract. Mix well.

3. Soak both sides of the protein bread with the mixture until thoroughly absorbed.

4. Place a nonstick skillet over medium flame and heat the butter. Swirl the butter to coat the base of the skillet.

5. Cook the french toast for 1 to 2 minutes per side, or until golden brown. Place on a plate and serve at once.

Cheesy Pancakes

Makes: 4 servings

Ingredients:

- ❖ Egg whites from 2 large eggs

- ❖ 2 oz grated cheddar cheese

- ❖ 1 garlic clove, minced

- ❖ 1 cup almond meal

- ❖ 1/2 tsp baking powder

- ❖ 2 Tbsp olive oil

- ❖ 1/4 cup filtered water

Instructions:

1. In a bowl, whisk the egg whites, then mix in the cheddar cheese, garlic, almond meal, baking powder, and filtered water.

2. Gradually drizzle in the olive oil as you whisk until thoroughly incorporated.

3. Place a nonstick skillet over medium high flame and coat with cooking spray.

4. Once the skillet is hot, ladle some of the mixture into the skillet to form a pancake. Cook on one side for about 1 minute or until bubbly. Flip over and cook for another 1 minute.

5. Stack on a plate and cook the remaining batter. Serve warm, preferably with butter or cream cheese.

Smoked Salmon Quiche

Makes: 6 servings

Ingredients:

- ❖ 9 oz smoked salmon
- ❖ 6 eggs
- ❖ 6 oz raw mushrooms
- ❖ 1 1/2 cups sliced leeks, white and pale green parts
- ❖ 3 Tbsp minced fresh thyme
- ❖ 2/3 cup chopped red pepper
- ❖ 2 1/4 cups unsweetened almond milk
- ❖ 1 1/2 tsp dry mustard
- ❖ 1 1/2 tsp paprika
- ❖ 3/4 tsp sea salt
- ❖ 3/4 tsp freshly ground black pepper
- ❖ 1/3 tsp cayenne pepper
- ❖ 1 1/2 cups crumbled goat cheese
- ❖ Coconut oil, for greasing

Instructions:

1. Set the oven to 375 degrees F to preheat.

2. Place a skillet over medium flame and heat a bit of coconut oil. Add the leeks and saute until tender. Once tender, stir in

the mushrooms and saute until partially tender. Add the peppers and season with salt, then saute for 4 minutes.

3. Sprinkle the thyme all over and stir quickly to combine, then remove from the heat. Set aside.

4. Prepare a small casserole or large pie plate. Crumble the smoked salmon into it, and then spread the leek mixture on top to form an even layer. Sprinkle the cheese over the top and then set aside.

5. In a bowl, whisk together the eggs, salt, cayenne, black pepper, milk, paprika, and mustard. Pour the mixture all over the ingredients in the casserole; do not stir.

6. Place the casserole in the oven and bake for 30 minutes. If the quiche is still uncooked in the center but browned around the edges, cover the casserole with aluminum foil and bake for an additional 25 to 30 minutes.

7. Remove the quiche out of the oven at the end of 50 minutes to an hour. Place on a wire rack to cool slightly, then slice and serve.

Special Raspberry Waffles

Makes: 4 waffles

Ingredients:

- ❖ 1 cup almond flour
- ❖ 2/3 cup coconut milk
- ❖ 4 Tbsp flaxseed meal
- ❖ 4 large eggs, beaten
- ❖ 2 tsp baking powder
- ❖ 2 tsp vanilla extract
- ❖ 4 Tbsp liquid stevia
- ❖ 1 cup fresh or frozen raspberries
- ❖ 1 1/2 Tbsp lemon juice
- ❖ Zest of 1/2 lemon
- ❖ 4 Tbsp grass fed butter
- ❖ 2 Tbsp stevia
- ❖ 6 oz double cream brie, sliced

Instructions:

1. In a bowl, combine the almond flour, flaxseed meal, baking powder, and liquid stevia. Stir in the eggs, coconut milk and vanilla extract until just combined; do not over-mix.

2. Prepare the waffle iron and cook based on manufacturer's directions.

3. Transfer the waffles to a plate and add the sliced brie on top. Set aside.

4. Place a nonstick skillet over medium flame and melt the butter.

5. Stir in the stevia until starting to brown, then stir in the raspberries, lemon juice, and lemon zest. Continue to stir as you cook until it turns into a jam consistency.

6. In a toaster oven, toast the waffles for 2 minutes, or until the brie is soft and waffles are crisp. Drizzle the raspberry mixture on top, then serve.

Baked Eggs on Avocado

Makes: 1 serving

Ingredients:

- ❖ 1 ripe avocado
- ❖ 2 fresh eggs
- ❖ 1/2 celery stalk, minced
- ❖ 1 small onion, minced
- ❖ 1/2 red bell pepper, seeded and chopped
- ❖ 1 tsp chopped fresh chives, parsley, or cilantro, for garnish
- ❖ Sea salt
- ❖ Freshly ground black pepper

Instructions:

1. Set the oven to 425 degrees F to preheat.

2. Halve the avocado and discard the seed. Scoop out about 3 tablespoons from the center of the avocado to create a pit for one egg per half.

3. Arrange the avocado on a baking sheet and set aside.

4. Carefully break the eggs open in two bowls, separating the yolks from the whites. Slip one yolk into each avocado pit, then add the white. Add the celery, onion, and bell pepper, then season with salt and pepper.

5. Bake the avocados for 15 minutes, or until eggs are cooked to a desired consistency. Sprinkle fresh herbs on top and serve at once.

Chapter 4 - Small Meals and Sides

Basic Bone Broth

Makes: 2 1/2 gallons

Ingredients:

- ❖ 1 lb organic chicken backbones
- ❖ 2 1/4 gallons filtered water
- ❖ 3 tsp coconut oil
- ❖ 1/2 bulb roasted garlic, peeled
- ❖ 3/4 cup roasted red onions, peeled
- ❖ 1 1/3 cup tomato paste from a glass jar
- ❖ 1 cup organic tomato pulp
- ❖ 3/4 cup sea salt
- ❖ 1 Tbsp freshly ground black pepper
- ❖ Optional: 4 Tbsp chopped fresh rosemary, 2 Tbsp cilantro with stems, and/or 2 Tbsp organic oregano

Instructions:

1. Place a 3 gallon pot over medium flame and heat the oil. Add the roasted garlic and onion and saute for 10 minutes.

2. Add the chicken backbones, tomato paste, tomato pulp, filtered water, sea salt, and black pepper. Stir in the herbs, if using.

3. Cover and set heat to lowest possible setting. Let simmer for 24 to 72 hours. Alternatively, use a slow cooker and cook half the batch or the amount that the cooker will allow. Long cooking time allows for a thicker and more nutrient dense broth.

4. After cooking, set the pot aside to cool to room temperature. Pour the broth through a sieve and discard the solids. Divide the broth into desired amounts based on personal preference and store in freezer containers. Refrigerate for up to 4 weeks or freeze for up to 4 months.

Tuna and Zucchini Roll-ups

Makes: 24 pieces

Ingredients:

- ❖ 3 medium zucchini
- ❖ 8 oz canned tuna, drained thoroughly
- ❖ 1 large avocado, peeled and pitted
- ❖ 3 Tbsp keto-friendly mayonnaise
- ❖ 3 tsp freshly squeezed lime juice
- ❖ 1 medium chili, seeded and minced
- ❖ Sea salt
- ❖ Freshly ground black pepper
- ❖ Cayenne pepper or paprika

Instructions:

1. Using a potato peeler, slice the zucchini lengthwise to create long ribbons. Slice the ribbons in half until you have about 24 pieces.

2. In a bowl, combine the tuna, mayonnaise, lime juice, and chili. Mash the avocado into the mixture, then season to taste with salt, pepper, and cayenne or paprika.

3. Spoon some of the tuna mixture to one end of each zucchini ribbon and roll up. Secure each roll with a toothpick. Serve at once.

Simple Seafood Soup

Makes: 2 servings

Ingredients:

- ❖ 4 oz peeled and deveined prawns
- ❖ 4 oz firm white fish fillet, cubed
- ❖ 2 Tbsp coconut oil
- ❖ 2 tomatoes, sliced
- ❖ 2 garlic cloves, mashed and peeled
- ❖ 1 red chili, sliced
- ❖ 1 leek, sliced
- ❖ 1/2 Tbsp fresh thyme
- ❖ 2 Tbsp white wine
- ❖ 2 1/4 liters filtered water
- ❖ Sea salt
- ❖ Freshly ground black pepper

Instructions:

1. Place a soup pot over medium flame and heat the oil. Once hot, stir in the celery and chili for 3 minutes, or until tender.

2. Add the water and white wine, then increase heat to a simmer.

3. Let simmer for 5 minutes, then carefully stir in the cubed fish fillet and prawns. Cook for 10 minutes, or until fish and prawns are cooked through.

4. Season to taste with salt and pepper, then stir in the thyme and serve at once.

Cheesy Chicken Sticks

Makes: 12 pieces

Ingredients:

- ❖ 1 lb chicken breast, free range
- ❖ 1 Tbsp chopped fresh thyme or parsley
- ❖ 1/2 tsp chili powder
- ❖ 1/2 cup grated Parmesan cheese
- ❖ 2 oz grass fed butter
- ❖ 2 garlic cloves, minced
- ❖ Sea salt
- ❖ Freshly ground black pepper

Instructions:

1. Set the oven to 350 degrees F to preheat. Coat a baking sheet with nonstick cooking spray and set aside.

2. Place a saucepan over medium flame and melt the butter. Saute the garlic until browned.

3. On a plate, combine the buttered garlic, thyme or parsley, chili powder, and Parmesan cheese.

4. Rinse and pat the chicken dry with paper towels. Slice into 12 long pieces, then coat with the cheese mixture.

5. Arrange the chicken pieces on the prepared baking sheet, then bake for 20 minutes, turning the pieces over halfway through the cooking time.

6. Once golden brown and cooked through, remove the chicken from the oven and set on a wire rack to cool slightly before serving.

Cauliflower Bites

Makes: 60 pieces

Ingredients:

- ❖ 1 large cauliflower
- ❖ 3 Tbsp grass fed butter
- ❖ 3 Tbsp heavy cream
- ❖ 3/4 cup grated strong cheddar cheese
- ❖ Egg whites from 6 fresh eggs
- ❖ Sea salt
- ❖ Freshly ground black pepper
- ❖ Paprika

Instructions:

1. Slice the cauliflower into florets and place in a saucepan. About 3 to 4 tablespoons of water and a dash of salt. Cook over medium flame until tender. Transfer to a food processor.

2. Add the butter and cream into the food processor and pulse until it achieves an oatmeal-like consistency. Season with salt and pepper.

3. Whisk the egg whites, preferably with an electric mixer, until stiff peaks form. Fold the cauliflower mixture into the egg whites, then refrigerate for at least half an hour.

4. Set the oven to 375 degrees F to preheat. Coat 2 large baking sheets with nonstick cooking spray.

5. Using a tablespoon, scoop the cauliflower mixture from the bowl and place on the prepared baking sheets. Bake for 20 minutes or until crisp and golden brown.

6. Sprinkle paprika over all the cauliflower bites and serve immediately.

Kimchi

Makes: 8 servings

Ingredients:

- ❖ 6 cups cold filtered water
- ❖ 1/4 cup sea salt
- ❖ 1 lb napa cabbage
- ❖ 4 oz daikon radish, peeled and julienned
- ❖ 2 scallions, ends trimmed, sliced into 1 inch bits
- ❖ 1 Tbsp minced garlic cloves
- ❖ 2 Tbsp peeled and minced fresh ginger root
- ❖ 2 3/4 cups Korean red pepper powder
- ❖ 2 Tbsp fish sauce

Instructions:

1. Slice the cabbage into bite sized pieces, removing the root end. Place the cabbage into a bowl and sprinkle in the salt, tossing to coat all pieces evenly.

2. Pour the cold water onto the cabbage until it is completely covered, adding more if needed. Cover the bowl with a plastic wrap or baking sheet and set aside from 12 to 24 hours; the longer, the better.

3. Sterilize a 2 liter glass jar with a tight lid and set aside.

4. Put a colander in your sink and drain the cabbage thoroughly, rinsing with cold water. Press any excess water out before placing in a bowl. Set aside.

5. In a larger bowl, combine the radish, scallions, garlic, ginger, red pepper powder, and fish sauce. Mix very well, then add the cabbage and toss everything with clean hands until the cabbage is completely coated in the sauce.

6. Transfer everything into the sterilized glass jar and seal tightly. Place on a cool and dark shelf and allow to ferment for 24 hours. The bubbles that will form in the mixture are normal.

7. Remove the lid from the jar and let the kimchi *breathe*, then seal again tightly. Refrigerate from 2 to 7 days before serving. Store in the refrigerator for up to 30 days.

Chapter 5 - Main Course

Sweet and Spicy Meatballs

Makes: 6 servings

Ingredients:

- ❖ 1 1/2 lb organic ground beef
- ❖ 1 1/2 lb organic ground pork
- ❖ 6 spring onions, chopped
- ❖ 3 large red chili peppers, chopped
- ❖ 2 tsp sea salt
- ❖ 2 tsp ginger powder
- ❖ 2 tsp garlic powder
- ❖ 4 Tbsp soy sauce
- ❖ 1/2 cup almond flour
- ❖ 2 Tbsp olive oil
- ❖ 2 Tbsp sesame oil
- ❖ 2/3 cup apricot preserves, no sugar added
- ❖ 1/3 cup filtered water
- ❖ 1/3 tsp red pepper flakes
- ❖ 3 Tbsp freshly squeezed lime juice

Instructions:

1. Combine the ground meat, spring onions, red chili peppers, salt, ginger and garlic powders, soy sauce, and almond flour in a bowl. Mix very well, then mold into meatballs; the smaller, the easier to cook.

2. Place a heavy bottom skillet over medium high flame and heat the olive and sesame oils. Cook the meatballs for 3 minutes per side or until cooked through and golden.

3. Meanwhile, place a small saucepan over medium flame and combine the apricot preserves, water, red pepper flakes, and lime juice. Bring to a boil, then reduce to a simmer. Stir frequently.

4. Arrange the meatballs on a platter and pour the sauce on top. Serve warm.

Slow Cooked Kelp Noodle Pesto

Makes: 2 servings

Ingredients:

- ❖ 6 oz kelp noodles
- ❖ 2 Tbsp coconut oil
- ❖ 2 Tbsp melted coconut or macadamia nut oil
- ❖ 1 cup packed fresh basil
- ❖ 2 Tbsp walnuts
- ❖ 2 garlic cloves
- ❖ 1 1/2 Tbsp fresh red chili
- ❖ 1 Tbsp lime juice
- ❖ 2 Tbsp freshly grated Parmesan cheese
- ❖ 1/6 tsp sea salt
- ❖ 1/8 tsp freshly ground black pepper

Instructions:

1. In a food processor, combine the basil, walnuts, garlic, coconut oil, lime juice, chili, salt, and pepper. Process until very smooth.

2. Place the kelp noodles in a 2 quart slow cooker and add the pesto. Toss to coat, then cover the slow cooker and cook for 3 to 4 hours on low, or until the kelp noodles become very tender.

3. Serve warm, preferably with lightly toasted protein bread.

Bell Pepper and Chicken Kebabs

Makes: 12 kebabs

Ingredients:

- ❖ 3 lb boneless and skinless chicken breasts
- ❖ 2 green bell peppers
- ❖ 2 red bell peppers
- ❖ 1 1/4 cups olive oil
- ❖ 5 garlic cloves, crushed
- ❖ Juice and zest of 1 1/2 lemons
- ❖ 1 1/2 Tbsp minced fresh parsley
- ❖ Sea salt
- ❖ Freshly ground black pepper

Instructions:

1. Soak 12 bamboo kebab skewers in salted water and set aside.

2. Slice the chicken breasts into 1 inch cubes.

3. In a bowl, combine the lemon zest, garlic, and 1/3 cup olive oil. Stir in the fresh parsley and season to taste with salt and pepper.

4. Add the cubed chicken into the marinade and turn several times to coat. Cover the bowl and refrigerate for 8 to 12 hours to marinate.

5. Remove the seeds from the bell peppers, then slice into 1 inch pieces. Set aside.

6. In a bowl, combine the remaining olive oil and lemon juice. Season to taste with salt and pepper.

7. Set the broiler to medium or prepare the grill.

8. Skewer the chicken cubes and peppers, then coat with the olive oil and lemon juice mixture. Broil for 10 minutes or until peppers are slightly charred and chicken is cooked through.

9. Arrange on a serving platter and serve.

Baked Scampi

Makes: 2 servings

Ingredients:

- ❖ 1/4 cup macadamia nut oil or grass fed butter
- ❖ 1 Tbsp chopped fresh parsley
- ❖ 1/2 Tbsp freshly squeezed lemon juice
- ❖ 1/2 Tbsp Dijon mustard
- ❖ 1/2 Tbsp chopped garlic cloves
- ❖ 6 oz kelp noodles
- ❖ 1/2 lb uncooked medium shrimp, peeled and deveined

Instructions:

1. Cook the kelp noodles based on package instructions. Place on a serving plate, cover with aluminum foil to keep warm, and set aside.

2. Set the oven to 450 degrees F to preheat.

3. Place a saucepan over medium flame and melt the butter or heat the oil. Add the mustard, garlic, parsley, and lemon juice. Stir well to combine or until butter or oil is melted. Turn off the heat.

4. Place the shrimp in a baking dish in a single layer. Pour the sauce all over, then bake for 12 minutes, or until the shrimp is cooked through.

5. Pour the sauce all over the kelp noodles and arrange the baked shrimp on top. Serve at once, preferably with protein bread.

Tuna Salad

Makes: 1 serving

Ingredients:

- ❖ 1/3 cup chunky light tuna in water, drained thoroughly
- ❖ 1 cup shredded lettuce
- ❖ 1 small tomato, diced
- ❖ 2 Tbsp chopped fresh mint
- ❖ 2 Tbsp chopped fresh parsley
- ❖ 1/2 green onion, sliced thinly
- ❖ 5 large kalamata olives, pitted
- ❖ 1/4 avocado, diced
- ❖ 1/2 small zucchini, sliced lengthwise
- ❖ 1/2 Tbsp balsamic vinegar
- ❖ 1/2 Tbsp extra virgin olive oil
- ❖ Sea salt
- ❖ Freshly ground black pepper

Instructions:

1. Place a nonstick skillet over medium flame and coat with nonstick cooking spray. Once very hot, grill the zucchini on both sides until slightly charred. Set aside to cool slightly.

2. Slice the zucchini into bite sized pieces, then toss into a salad bowl with the lettuce, tomatoes, tuna, mint, parsley, green onion, olives, and avocado.

3. In a bowl, whisk together the balsamic vinegar and olive oil. Season to taste with salt and pepper.

4. Drizzle the dressing all over the salad and toss to coat. Serve at once.

Spaghetti Bolognese

Makes: 6 servings

Ingredients:

- ❖ 1/2 Tbsp coconut oil
- ❖ 12 oz kelp noodles
- ❖ 2 oz diced pancetta or bacon
- ❖ 1/3 cup diced celery
- ❖ 1/2 cup chopped yellow onion
- ❖ 1 bay leaf
- ❖ 1/2 Tbsp minced garlic
- ❖ 1/2 tsp sea salt
- ❖ 1/4 tsp freshly ground black pepper
- ❖ 1 1/2 Tbsp fresh oregano
- ❖ 1 1/2 Tbsp fresh thyme
- ❖ 2 Tbsp fresh parsley
- ❖ 1/4 tsp ground nutmeg
- ❖ 1/4 tsp ground cinnamon
- ❖ 1/4 lb ground organic liver
- ❖ 1/2 lb grass fed ground beef
- ❖ 1/4 lb organic ground pork or pork sausage with casings removed
- ❖ 1/2 cup bone broth

- 1 cup tomato sauce from a glass jar

- 2 cups crushed tomatoes, undrained

- 1/4 tsp stevia glycerite

- Optional: 2 Tbsp organic heavy cream, 1 Tbsp organic butter, and/or 1/2 cup freshly grated Parmesan cheese

Instructions:

1. Rinse the kelp noodles under cold running water, then drain thoroughly. Place the kelp noodles inside a 3 quart slow cooker and add water until covered. Cover and cook for 3 hours on low, or until al dente. Drain thoroughly and set aside.

2. In the meantime, place a medium saucepan over medium high flame and heat the coconut oil. Cook the bacon until almost browned, then set to the side of the saucepan.

3. Add the onion and celery to the pan and cook until tender. Stir in the garlic, oregano, thyme, nutmeg, cinnamon, bay leaf, salt, and pepper. Saute until fragrant.

4. Reduce heat to low, then stir in the beef, liver, and pork. Saute for about 6 minutes or until meat is cooked through.

5. Stir in the tomato sauce and cook for 2 minutes, stirring constantly. Scrape the bottom of the pan to loosen any browned bits. Continue to cook until mixture is thickened.

6. Stir in the broth and the tomatoes with their juices. Increase heat to a boil.

7. Once boiling, reduce to a simmer and cook for 30 minutes or until thickened, stirring occasionally.

8. Stir in the butter and cream, if using, and simmer for 3 minutes. Remove the bay leaf and season with salt and pepper to taste, if desired. Turn off the heat and cover until kelp noodles are ready.

9. Add the cooked kelp noodles to the sauce and mix well to combine. Sprinkle Parmesan cheese all over, then serve.

Pork and Mushroom Meatballs

Makes: 6 servings

Ingredients:

- ❖ 2 1/2 lb organic ground pork
- ❖ 15 dried shiitake mushrooms
- ❖ 2 Tbsp soy sauce
- ❖ 1/2 tsp garlic powder
- ❖ 1 tsp sea salt
- ❖ 1/2 tsp freshly ground black pepper
- ❖ 1 tsp granulated Splenda
- ❖ 4 Tbsp chopped green onions
- ❖ 2 eggs
- ❖ 1 tsp sesame oil

Instructions:

1. Boil 2 cups of water in a small pot over medium flame, then add the mushrooms. Boil for 5 minutes, then turn off the heat and cover. Set aside for 20 minutes.

2. Remove the mushrooms using a slotted spoon and press out excess liquid. Discard the tough stems, then mince.

3. In a bowl, combine the ground pork, soy sauce, garlic powder, sea salt, pepper, Splenda, green onion, sesame oil, and mushrooms. Mix well.

4. Add the egg and knead into the mixture until thoroughly combined.

5. Boil a pot of water over medium high flame. Using a teaspoon, scoop about 2 teaspoonfuls of the meat mixture into your hands and mold into meatballs.

6. Drop the meatballs into the pot of water and boil for about 8 to 10 minutes, or until meatballs are cooked through.

7. Remove with a slotted spoon and serve.

Chapter 6 - Snacks and Desserts

Coconut and Cinnamon Balls

Makes: 15 pieces

Ingredients:

- ❖ 1 1/2 cups coconut milk
- ❖ 1 1/2 cups coconut butter
- ❖ 1 1/2 cups shredded coconut
- ❖ 1 1/2 tsp Splenda
- ❖ 1 1/2 tsp vanilla extract
- ❖ 2/3 tsp cinnamon
- ❖ 2/3 tsp nutmeg

Instructions:

1. Pour water into a small double boiler. Alternatively, pour water into a saucepan and place a glass bowl on top of it to make a small double boiler.

2. Combine the coconut milk and butter, Splenda, vanilla extract, cinnamon and nutmeg in the bowl and place over medium flame.

3. Stir constantly until all the ingredients are fully combined and the butter has melted. Turn off the heat.

4. Set the bowl aside for 5 minutes to slightly cool, then transfer into the refrigerator. Chill for at least half an hour.

5. Take the bowl out of the fridge and use a spoon to scoop the mixture out and form balls about 1 inch in size.

6. Spread the shredded coconut on a plate and roll the balls to coat. Arrange the balls on a platter and refrigerate for at least one hour to become firm.

7. Serve chilled and store excess in the refrigerator.

Chocolate Mint Bars

Makes: 24 pieces

Ingredients:

- ❖ 2 1/4 cups almond flour
- ❖ 1/2 cup and 3 Tbsp granulated sugar substitute
- ❖ 1/3 cup unsweetened cocoa powder
- ❖ 5 oz dark chocolate (90 percent cocoa solids)
- ❖ 6 oz melted butter
- ❖ 2/3 tsp xanthan gum
- ❖ 2/3 tsp baking powder
- ❖ 1/3 tsp sea salt
- ❖ 1/3 cup almond oil
- ❖ 2 medium eggs, beaten
- ❖ 2 1/4 tsp peppermint extract

Instructions:

1. Set the oven to 375 degrees F to preheat. Line a baking sheet with baking paper and set aside.

2. In a bowl, combine the cocoa powder, almond flour, 1/2 cup sweetener, salt, baking powder, and xanthan gum.

3. In another bowl, combine 1 1/2 tsp peppermint extract, beaten egg, almond oil, and butter.

4. Combine the egg mixture into the flour mixture and stir well until you form a dough. Knead the dough until smooth, then shape into a flat rectangle.

5. Transfer the dough onto the prepared baking sheet and bake for 25 minutes, or until firm. Set on a wire rack to cool, then slice into 24 bars.

6. Set oven to 250 degrees F and place the baking sheet back inside. Bake for 15 minutes, then turn the bars over and bake for an additional 15 minutes.

7. Turn off the oven heat and let the bars stand inside the oven until cooled.

8. Melt the chocolate in a double boiler and stir in the remaining peppermint extract and sweetener.

9. Remove the bars from the oven and drizzle the chocolate mixture on top. Set aside to let the chocolate topping set before serving.

Mocha and Vanilla Butter Pops

Makes: 12 single servings

Ingredients:

- ❖ 1/2 cup coconut oil

- ❖ 1/2 cup grass fed butter

- ❖ 1/4 cup heavy cream

- ❖ 2 Tbsp cocoa powder

- ❖ 1 tsp coffee extract

- ❖ 1/2 cup Splenda

Instructions:

1. Place the butter in a bowl and set aside at room temperature for 5 minutes or microwave for 10 seconds to soften.

2. Stir the Splenda, cocoa powder, coffee extract, and coconut oil into the butter and set aside to cool if the butter is warm from the microwave. Combine very well, preferably with an electric mixer, and set aside.

3. Line 12 mini muffin tins with paper liners.

4. Divide the heavy cream mixture among the prepared muffin tins to form a cream layer. Refrigerate for 15 minutes, or until firm.

5. Take the muffin tins out of the refrigerator and pour the mocha mixture evenly into each tin. Stick a small popsicle stick into the center of each piece.

6. Place the muffin tins in the freezer and freeze for at least half an hour. Serve frozen and store excess in the freezer.

Butter Pumpkin Balls

Makes: 2 servings

Ingredients:

- ❖ 1/2 cup grass fed butter
- ❖ 4 Tbsp refined coconut oil
- ❖ 1 cup pureed pumpkin
- ❖ 1/8 tsp each: cinnamon, nutmeg, clove, ginger
- ❖ 1/4 to 1/2 tsp Splenda

Instructions:

1. Melt the coconut oil in a small saucepan over low flame or in the microwave until liquid. Stir the butter into it, mixing well with a fork until completely combined.

2. Whip the pureed pumpkin into the mixture until you get a smooth and creamy consistency. Stir in the cinnamon, nutmeg, clove, ginger, and Splenda.

3. Line a baking tray with parchment paper and drop the mixture onto it with about a tablespoon per piece.

4. Refrigerate the baking tray for at least 15 minutes or until the pieces are firm.

5. Take the tray out of the mixture and roll each piece into ball shapes about 1 inch in size. Return to the tray and refrigerate for at least one hour. Serve chilled and store excess in the refrigerator.

Coconut and Blueberry Mini Cakes

Makes: 10 servings

Ingredients:

- ❖ 1/4 cup grass fed butter
- ❖ 1/3 cup coconut oil
- ❖ 1/2 cup fresh or frozen blueberries
- ❖ 2 oz cream cheese, softened
- ❖ 2 Tbsp coconut cream
- ❖ 1/2 tsp Splenda

Instructions:

1. Place a saucepan over low flame, then stir in the coconut oil and butter. Stir until thoroughly combined, then turn off the heat and set aside for 5 minutes.

2. Once the butter and coconut oil mixture have cooled slightly, stir in the cream cheese, coconut cream, and Splenda.

3. Transfer the mixture to a dish, then fold in the blueberries and mix well to combine.

4. Place the dish in the freezer and freeze for at least 1 hour, or until firm. Serve chilled and store excess in the freezer.

Here's a Preview of our Books:

Body Language: Learn How to Read and Understand People, Master Your Social Skills, Business Meetings and Romantic Encounters!

This book contains proven steps and strategies on how to understand people and how to interact with them wisely without having to question your own personality and conscious acts when faced with challenging instances. If you have questions, clarifications, or even any doubt as regards your own actions or how you see yourself treat other people, you don't need to fret! It is just normal. Take for instance a job interview which you have been preparing for about a week. You dress up properly: the perfect pair of well-shined shoes, right coat, right plain and not-so-skinny tie; you have every document you need that could validate you well as a candidate; you speak fluently, about three to four languages maybe; you have the right manners, as well as your perfectly shaped smile. But they didn't call you back—for about four months now.

What went wrong? Was it your documents? - That they didn't find the one skill they might have been looking for? Was it your tie? Would it have changed the result if you went with the checkered and skinny one? You try to rewind the facts that happened during that interview and you find no flaw. But you overlooked how your body language was delivered. You forgot to pinpoint some bodily movements or gestures that might have led the interviewer into a wrong place, into a wrong idea of you.

See, this is only one simple situation. If you really look into it, there is some intricacy weaved in that situation, an intricacy that might not be so complex after all - if you had only known. Body language is not only body movement. There is much about it and like everything else ever known to be existent in this world, there is science to it. As you read through the pages of this book, body language would no longer be a dubious concern for you anymore.

You can check/download the book from <u>HERE</u>.

HTML: Step by Step Beginners Guide to HTML

*The book "**HTML: Step by Step Beginners Guide to HTML**" will provide all essential information and training during the book which you'll need in order to upgrade your skills later with other languages and even with more sophisticated HTML.*

The reason why we start our "Learn Web Design" series with HTML is because he is the core to every website out there. No matter how basic or sophisticated one website is the HTML is always there and is essential for its existence.

In order to perfectly understand the material we'll go through everything from the absolute beginning. We'll do some exercises because the only way to master programming is by constant exercise and learning.

All the material in this book can be learned in less than a day but exercising and upgrading your skills later on is essential to becoming a good programmer.

You can check/download the book from <u>HERE</u>.

Ketogenic Diet: The Easiest Way to Lose Weight Fast for Beginners with Low-Carb, High-Fat Keto Clarity Diet!

Do you want to lose weight fast enough for a special event? Are you eager to jump-start weight loss so that you can get motivated? You might like to consider the ketogenic diet!

The keto diet is an extremely low carb and high fat diet that takes advantage of ketosis, which is a state that causes the body to burn stored fat. To trigger ketosis, one must eliminate carbohydrates and start consuming fat to train the body to burn fat instead of glucose for energy. This might seem like a dream come true, but it is quite a challenging diet to follow.

The good news is that this book will guide you through the keto diet. You will find a 7 day keto meal plan to make things easy for you, along with the recipes for each meal of the day. All the recipes call for cheap and healthy ingredients that are guaranteed to give you energy and designed to bring your body into a state of ketosis.

Enjoy the benefits of a strong and lean body. The keto diet can help you to lose weight, gain more energy, and improve your overall health.

You can check/download the book from *HERE*

Long Distance Relationships: Learn how to keep the fire! Improve your relationship and make it last!

In this book I've written the primary ideas and advices about how you should behave and engage to your significant other. Here I've pointed out not only once that the distance in between people can only make them stronger they are really committed and after all it's only just the beginning of something new, concerning your future life together. Pureness and emotional connection will only reveal people's true intentions and their worthiness of your presence, affection and attention. If you're in a situation like that and dead sure in your emotional commitment to that special someone this book is for you. I've presented one of the simplest coping mechanisms. If you're willing your love life will be thrilling and exciting and everything will be worth it in the end.

You can check/download the book from HERE

Quit Smoking: Easiest Way to Stop Smoking for Life

For years I've been smoking two packs a day, ignoring the cry for help coming from my body.

I was a promising young athlete when I slipped. In the beginning I felt cooler smoking with the other kids. It was like the social boost, so desperately needed for a kid on my age back then. Years passed, my lung capacity decreased and as you can guess my athlete years came to an end.

Truth is… at the beginning it was all about the social status. Being with the other popular kids pretending to be something more than the others felt like the right thing to do at that moment. And like most of my decisions from my childhood I made a mistake. For years I've been saying to myself every night "I will quit smoking from tomorrow" and as you can guess it's not that easy.

From the moment that the thought about not smoking anymore gets in your head the anxiety hits you like a train. I couldn't stop the thoughts about smoking and how good would I feel from invading my mind. I've tried numerous amounts of different pills, gums and all sort of mambo jambo without any success.

There are generally three types of people that can manage to quit smoking for real.

- The really strong personalities. Those are the people that grab life in their own hands and turn the wheel when It's needed.
- The scared people. Those are the ones that in most cases had a word with the doctor and they finally heard the words that we all read on the cigar packs. Unfortunately if you get to that point it's probably too late.
- And there's the 3rd group of people – the carrying ones. Most of you know that the passive smoke that we exhale is just as dangerous for our loving ones around us, as the one we inhale. So if we're not concerned about our own wellbeing,

finding someone important and special to give you the motivation is a good way to start.

Think about it. If you're ready to take the big step of living a longer and healthier life, in which group would you put yourself?

Quitting smoking isn't easy but it all depends on you, on that what you want for yourself, for your close ones and for everyone around you.

If you continue reading you'll get a whole new perspective of the world without smoking. The key to quit them once and for all and most importantly you'll have more years to live and make your family and friends happy.

You can check/download the book from <u>HERE</u>

Subscribe for FREE Kindle Books

<u>Click here to subscribe to our list and start receiving Free Kindle Books in your inbox.</u>

Conclusion

Thank you again for downloading this book!

I hope this book was able to help you to begin the keto clarity diet and achieve your fitness goals.

The next step is to form the habit of planning and preparing your meals ahead of time. You should also sign up for an aerobic and strength exercise program to become healthy and make the keto clarity diet work for you.

Finally, if you enjoyed this book, then I'd like to ask you for a favor, would you be kind enough to leave a review for this book on Amazon? It'd be greatly appreciated!